The Lady Oasis Healing Experience

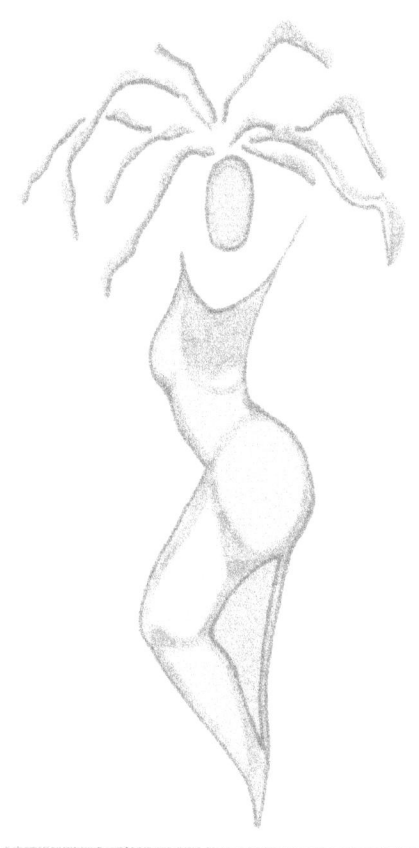

Written by Mildred 'Missie' Shealey

The Lady Oasis Healing Experience: A Guide to Wholistic Healing For Women

Written by Mildred 'Missie' Shealey

This booklet is intended for educational and informational purposes only. Before starting the Lady Oasis Natural Healing Experience, please see a qualified healthcare professional if you have questions about your health.

Published by:
Mildred 'Missie' Shealey
Sandy Springs, GA 30350

Website: www.ladyoasis.ning.com
Email: ladyoasis@gmail.com

Table of Contents

Dedication

I dedicate this book to my mother Helen Elizabeth Leggette. As a child, I often saw her intensely reading a bright orange book that I now know today to have been the Back To Eden book by Jethro Kloss. She often used natural remedies to cure and maintain herself and her eight children. She also picked and served fresh vegetables from her two gardens and utilized vinegar water castor oil and 'elephant leaves' on a regular basis. I thank her for unknowingly protecting and sustaining me into adulthood, even before I officially arrived. Thank you mom, I love you unconditionally!

Introduction

The Lady Oasis Natural Healing Experience is a plethora of accumulated research that was created some 13 years ago as a reference for friends and family to use at their leisure to aid in suggestions on natural healing methods explored basically through the utilization of simple foods, pure water, regular eliminations, green supplements, and a healthy state of mind and environment. It was originally called *Lady Oasis: A Wholistic Guide to Healing* but was recently updated a book format, enhanced, and prepared with more exciting details for women to use for themselves as well as share with friends and family!

The heart of this book is to guide you into a new beginning of self. Overall intent here is to introduce a lifestyle of vigor with boundless possibilities for health. There are a multitude of road maps serving as guides towards natural health and yet each person is different in the path required for their personal health. Given the variety of options widely available, I thank you for choosing Lady Oasis.

The Lady Oasis Natural Healing Experience is what I know to be true for me in my path towards a better and healthier self and I wish the same to manifest for you in your similar quest for optimal health.

In advance I wholeheartedly say, Happy Healing!

About the Author

Mildred (Missie) Shealey, is originally from Pittsburgh, Pennsylvania and has lived in the Metropolitan D.C. area. She currently resides in Atlanta Georgia and has been there since 1996. She attended Paine College in Augusta, GA and is a graduate of the Art Institute of Pittsburgh.

Ms. Shealey has spent over 15 years of her professional career as a topnotch Wardrobe Specialist for high-end retailers such as St. John's Boutique, Neiman Marcus, Nordstrom, Calvin Klein and Saks Fifth Avenue. She is also a contributing writer for the Onyx Woman Magazine, online.

A major accomplishment for Ms. Shealey was having her children's storybook published entitled, *Pookie Lookie: The Pink Spotted Panda Bear*, which through engaging colorful illustration teaches children about the importance of love and self-acceptance. In preparing future generations, Missie is also teaching her daughter, Janiyah, the importance of healthy choices as she similarly embraces healthier lifestyle choices amidst her interaction with the vast world around her.

For well over 20 years Ms. Shealey has researched, incorporated and widely shared her findings on Natural Health with immediate family, friends, and co-workers.

In addition she is also a Certified Reflexologist. Her goal within the following pages is to share her healthy findings with beginners who are looking for the path towards a healthier well-being. Missie has spent the first half of her life enjoying a career helping people look good on the outside. Now she would like to dedicate the next phase of her journey helping people to feel good on the inside.

Thank you for choosing to be Fierce, Fabulous and ready to Heal!

Testimonies

"Thank you for Blessing Edwin and I with your book in January to help make 2011 a great year for us!
    --- Lesans 'Soni' Heard Montgomery - Pittsburgh, PA

REMOVE

My first chapter is called Remove. This is where I like to say, all the 'fun' begins. So here we go!

First:
Go through your refrigerator and get rid of all foods that have one or more of the following ingredients as the first five ingredients:

> A. ENRICHED
> B. HYDROGENATED
> C. SALT
> D. SUGAR
> E. HIGH FRUCTOSE SYRUP

Next:
Remove all white products, unless you have white nut milks, fruits or veggies and water. Now, do the same in your pantry and your cupboards. Great! You will probably have nothing left EXCEPT fruits or veggies and water.

VERY GOOD! Now we are on the right track!!

Finally:
Let's get rid of all meats (YES, EVEN YOUR STEAK!)
Great job! Now, that wasn't too painless right?!

REPLACE

My second chapter is called **REPLACE**.
This chapter will give you your main staple items to get you started towards the 'NEW' you. It so exciting but also challenging so please don't beat yourself up. Always remember that life is a never ending journey. Sit back, relax and enjoy the ride.

First:
Fill your refrigerator to the brim with the following fresh items:

A. LOTS OF YOUR FAORITE ORGANIC FRUITS AND VEGETABLES
B. LOTS OF DISTILLED WATER
C. ORGANIC GREEN, LEAFY VEGGIES
D. FRESH WILD SALMON,TILAPIA OR SNAPPER
E. GARLIC, ONIONS, BEAN SPROUTS, CILANTRO AND FRESH GINGER,
F. ALMOND OR RICE MILK

Fill your pantry and cupboards with the following items:

A. OATMEAL,
B. RAW HONEY, AGAVE NECTAR
C. DRY BEANS, BROWN RICE,
D. NUTS – CASHEW, WALNUT, BRAZILIAN, ALMOND AND PECAN
E. EXTRA VIRGIN OLIVE OIL AND COCONUT OIL
F. RAW APPLE CIDER VINEGAR (BRAGGS)
G. NATURAL HERBAL TEAS - PEPPERMINT, SPEARMINT, CHAMOMILE, CHAI, ETC
H. DRY SPICES

Buy a good juicer, food processor, blender and medium storage containers for food.
Also Purchase Barley green essentials (powdered form)and Epsom salt (detox baths)

Purchase the following herbs in capsule liquid or powder form,

A. CAYENNE PEPPER-for circulation
B. GOLDEN SEAL-a natural antibiotic
C. VITAMIN C-builds immune system
D. RED RASPBERRY- strengthens the women's reproductive system
E. CASCARA SAGRADA- for regular bowel movements
F. PSYLLIUM HUSK AND POWDERED FLAX SEED- additional bulking agents
   for the colon
G. GOTU KOLA- memory and concentration
H. COD LIVER OIL- internal lubrication and great health benefits

RECHARGE

On your mark, Get Ready, Get Set, **HEAL**!

I named this chapter **RECHARGE** because that is exactly what we are aiming to do, **RECHARGE** our Bodies, Minds and Spirits, one mango at a time. (my favorite fruit)

Morning routine:

Enjoy a 8 oz of water with juice of one lemon(half is ok too) before you do anything else. This will help to get your digestive juices to flowing 30 -45 minutes later, take 4 psyllium husk capsules. Drink with 8.oz of water. EXTREMELY IMPORTANT! Did I say EXTREMELY IMPORTANNT? Oh, ok.

Mid –morning breakfast
Drink a cup of hot jasmine tea (my favorite tea) or tea of choice and add to it a half a tsp of coconut oil and agave nectar or honey to taste. Relax and take the morning in.
Prepare a Green Machine smoothie (see recipe) and add a teaspoon of barley green essentials. Blend until frothy and creamy. Enjoy
If you still need a little something extra, you can prepare a bowl of oatmeal and add cinnamon (add to water first) raisins (for sweetener) walnuts (optional) and almond milk (for creaminess)

Lunch
Eat a HUGE green salad with or without a small portion of salmon on the side. Add freshly prepared salad dressing. Add walnuts and orange flavored cranberries,

Enjoy!
Drink water, lemonade or tea,
Keep it simple

Dinner

Large salad. Get creative! You have tons of veggies to choose from
(Use same dressing recipe)
Roasted veggies of choice.
Hot tea with a twist of lemon.

Dessert options
A nice bowl of your favorite 'juicy' fruit (mango would be my choice)

OR

¼ Almonds, ¼ unsalted sunflower seeds, ¼ raisins or cranberries all mixed together. Blend with 8 figs in a food processor. Roll into balls. Enjoy!!

OR

If you have food processor, blend two cups of frozen fruit with 3tbs of fresh apple juice, a tsp of REAL vanilla extract, a dab of honey. Blend to a sorbet consistency. Enjoy!!

Exercise, Exercise, Exercise

You cannot receive long lasting and life changing benefits with healthy foods alone.

You must exercise your temple and get the blood flowing, the mind excited and the soul invigorated! Let's go!

Here are some basic options for you to consider. If nothing else, just WALK!

1. Walk daily for 30 minutes. (EXTREMELY IMPORTANT!!!)

2. Weight train 3x a week - strengthens the muscles

3. Do yoga- strengthens the mind and body

4. Kick boxing- strengths the body and keeps the heart happy

5. Pole dancing – keeps the body strong and the mind excited.(I heard it was the new 'IN' thing in the exercise world!)

RELAX

This is so important, always find time to relax, no matter what I know it can be almost impossible but it is so necessary. Stress is not your friend and if your not careful it can take your life away from you. If it gets too heavy, stop and ask yourself these question: What's the worst case scenario? Will it matter five years from know?

Answer the questions honestly, accept the answers and KEEP IT MOVING!

Here's my favorite part of the day. After I put my daughter to bed and take off my 'mommy hat', if I'm not too exhausted, I escape!

Here are some of my relaxation techniques:

Rejuvenate
Take a nice hot bubble bath everyday, if possible, but at least twice a week.

Add a half a cup of Epsom salt to relax sore muscles to detox the body and mind.

Light a scented candle soak for at least 30 minutes.

Lubricate with warm coconut

Or almond oil. (don't go to bed dry and ashy ladies!) Wash your face with the gel from the aloe vera leaf. Or a natural cleanser of choice. Add coconut oil to moisturize while you sleep.(a little goes along way)

A little extra- For 'Fun Fridays', add a cup of powdered milk and two tablespoons of raw cacao powder to running bath water with your choice of fragrant free bubble bath. Enjoy just for the heck of it!

Enjoy

Indulge in a hot cup of peppermint or chamomile tea with a dollop of honey and a squirt of fresh lemon juice. If you really need to relax and two bags of tea.

Right before bedtime: Take two capsules of cascara sagrada with a small glass of water. Do this nightly for two weeks. This is a safe, natural stimulant but as advised ALWAYS check with your doctor and do some research for your own comfort. This is the only laxative that I take, when needed.

Some more sound advice to heed to:

Eliminate negative self- talk. Unfortunately we can be our worst critics and we are slowly talking ourselves into depression and self doubt. STOP IT!

Do something wonderful just for yourself. Buy your self some flowers or take yourself to a movie or by some sexy pumps to go with your new ATTITUDE!
We love shoes!

Listen to only positive music. Stay away from negative people.

Hopefully they don't live in your house!
BE GENTLE WITH YOUR SELF AND STAY CALM.
Find your place of peace, where ever it is. Journal, write all about YOU because YOU are INDEED important.

Talk to your creator, your life source. Find your HAPPINESS.

CHANT, PRAY OR MEDITATE. Just BE!

REJOICE

Congratulations in advance for finding the True YOU again!

PRACTICE THIS FOR THE NEXT 90 DAYS!

Prepare for the healing process in advance by eating huge salads and drinking lots of water to get your body ready for the anticipated 'Healing Experience'.

1. Make a list of your ailments prior to starting your healing journey.

2. Take a before picture when you began. After 30 days take a picture, after 60 days take a picture and after 90 days take a picture of yourself .

3. Purchase a gorgeous journal and begin to write about your thoughts and feeling, daily.

4. Take a daily morning enema of warm water for the first two weeks help flush the toxins from your body.

5. It is highly recommend to get a professional colonic at least once a month for the next 3 months. Two colonics monthly would be ideal. Find a therapist that comes highly recommended and be sure that they to use disposal equipment.

Remember Ladies, This is a slow and gradual awakening. If you have never done this before, be GENTLE with yourself.

If you experience a HEALING CRISIS (headaches, nausea, dizziness), drink lots of water and vegetable juices. Relax. If severe, lease contact your doctor IMMEDIATELY.

RECIPES

Basic Breakfast recipes

<u>Ambrosia fruit bowl</u>

This recipe is very easy, tasty and so good for you.

1 cup of blueberries
1 cup of chopped granny smith apples
I cup of sliced strawberries
I ripened banana, thinly sliced
I cup of sliced grapes
I cup of sliced juicy oranges
¼ cup of orange juice (freshly squeezed)
½ cup of grated coconut
½ cup of chopped walnuts
1 tablespoon of cinnamon
3 tablespoons of agave nectar
Mix all ingredients in a large bowl.
Chill. Serve. Enjoy

Sweet and Spicy Oatmeal

This is a nice twist on plain oatmeal.

2 cups of Almond milk
1 cup of raw oatmeal
½ tsp of cinnamon
½ tsp of flaxseed powder
2 tbsp of blueberries
Walnuts (optional)
1 tbsp of agave nectar or honey

Prepare raw oatmeal according to direction
But instead of water use almond milk (bring to a slight boil)
Add cinnamon and agave nectar or honey to the milk.
Continue following directions until done.
Put oatmeal into a serving bowl. Add flaxseed powder and stir.
Top with blueberries and walnuts. Enjoy!

Peach cobbler smoothie
It tastes like a real old fashioned peach cobbler

2 Cup of frozen peaches
2 cups of organic peach nectar
2 handfuls of raw baby spinach
2 ripened banana
½ cup of uncooked raw oats
½ tsp of cinnamon
½ tsp of nutmeg

Put all ingredients in a blender and puree for I minute
Enjoy!

Green machine smoothie
(**Missie's favorite smoothie**)
2 cups of fresh apple juice (Simply Apple is a good brand)
2 ripened bananas with brown spots (very important)
2 large handfuls of raw baby spinach
1 pinch of fresh cilantro PINCH OF FRESH CILANTRO
3 beet root leaves
2 cups of frozen mixed fruit
¼ cup of raw oatmeal
¼ cup of powdered flaxseed
½ teaspoon of cinnamon
Put all ingredients into a blender
Blend for 1 minute until creamy. Enjoy!

Lunch recipes

For lunch I recommend large salads.
These are the selected ingredients that you should include.
You can do a combination of any of your favorites and
make the happiest salad ever. Or be daring and use them
all. Either way, you are sure to be pleased, healthy
And happy!

Green, Green salad

Romaine lettuce
Thinly sliced red onions
Sliced cucumbers
Shredded carrots
Cherry tomatoes, sliced in half
Cilantro
Sliced avocados
Chopped green apples
Raisins
Walnuts
Sunflower seeds
Sprouts
yellow or red peppers
baby spinach
arugula.
radishes
sun dried tomatoes

Salad dressing recipe

This is a basic recipe for an easy and tasty salad dressing. You can get creative and add your own seasonings according to your taste buds.

Juice of whole lemon
2 tbsp of honey or agave nectar
½ tsp of Dry basil
3 tablespoons of extra virgin olive oil
Blend all ingredients together. Add sparingly to salad. Enjoy!

Yummy Lettuce wraps
These wraps are, quick easy and addictive

Large romaine lettuce leafs
Scoop of Hummus of choice
Handful of Sprouts
4 cherry tomatoes, sliced
2 Basil leafs
Thinly sliced red onion, to taste
Tbsp of raisins (optional for a sweet surprise)

Wash and dry lettuce leaves
Spread generous amount of hummus on leaf
Layer with remaining ingredients.
Fold in sides and roll leaf from bottom until completely
Closed. Enjoy!

Dinner Time

BAKED SALMON

6 OZ SALMON
4 tbsp of crushed garlic
2 tbsp of crush fresh ginger root
Juice of one lemon
3 tbsp of raw honey, pure maple syrup, or agave nectar
3 tbsp of coconut oil

1. Mix all ingredients except salmon
2. Place salmon in a baking dish
3. Pour marinade over salmon, covering evenly. Refrigerate up to three hrs or overnight
4. In a pre-heated 375 degree oven, bake salmon covered for 15
5. Serve with a fresh green salad and baked veggies.

GRILLED VEGGIES

1 large red onion, cut into chunks
1 of each, red and yellow peppers, cut into chunks
1 cup of cherry tomatoes, sliced in half
3 tbsp of olive oil
1 tbsp of Italian seasonings

1. Preheat oven to 350
2. Mix all ingredients together with olive oil and place in a baking pan

3. Bake in oven for 25 minutes or until veggies are tender, enjoy!

<u>Old Fashion Lemonade with a jolt</u>
This is a refreshing lemonade that will excite your senses!

Juice of 6 lemons
6 cups of distilled water
1 cup of freshly squeezed ginger root juice
2 tbsp of fresh anise
Honey or agave nectar, to taste

Bring water honey or agave, and anise to a boil. Remove from heat.
Let sit for five minutes
Add remaining ingredients and stir.

Serve warm in the winter and over ice in the summer. Enjoy!

REFERENCES

These are a few of my favorite books to read and websites to explore:

1. *Prescription for Nutritional Healing* - James Balch

2. *The Juice Man's Power of Juicing* - Jay Kordich

3. *Anti -Aging Manual* -Joseph Marion

4. *Heal Thyself* – Queen Afua

5. *Sacred Woman* – Queen Afua

6. *The Tropical Spa* - Sophie Benge

7. *The Complete Book Of Juicing* – Michael T. Murray

8. *Raw Food, A Complete Guide for Every Meal of the Day* - Erica Palmcrantz

9. http://rawfoodrehab.ning.com

10. http://www.greensmoothiequeen.com/

11. http://www.karynraw.com/

12. http://www.womengoraw.com/

13. http://www.reversediabetesin30days.com/

14. http://www.foodincmovie.com/spread-the-word.php

CONGRATULATIONS IN ADVANCE!
Continue to love YOU, and your FABULOUS SELF!

Love, your healing experience coach,

Missie Shealey

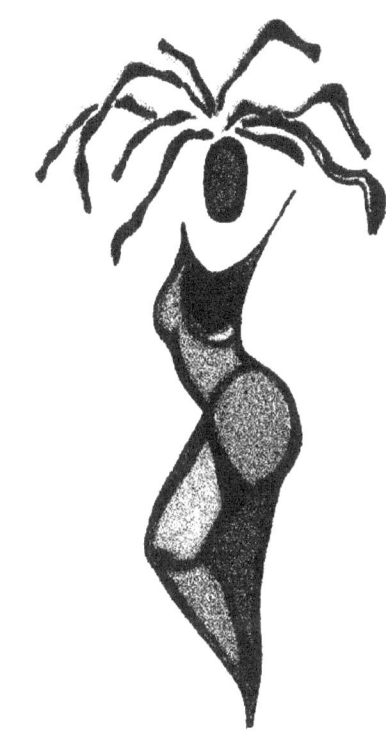

STAY FABULOUS!